1

Table of Contents

Introduction

There are quite a few books on the internet about nutrition and diets for kids with ADHD or ADD (attention deficit). I have found them to be informative but a little general in nature. In this book I am going to go over some specific recipes and meals that in my opinion will help kids with attention deficit and/or a hyperactivity problem. The recipes and meals that I outline below are meant to provide nutrition for a growing kid while at the same time reducing ingredients that can make ADHD worse and increasing ingredients that can make ADHD better. This particular article is going to focus on "smoothies and shakes". The goal of these meal plans and recipes is not weight loss so they can still taste good and filling. In fact, if your child is on medication you are going to need to feed them meals that will keep their weight up not down. This fact makes meal planning a lot easier than if you are also trying to lose weight.

ADHD is a neurological condition that impacts executive function, working memory, impulsivity, focus, distractibility, and emotional health. Here, learn about ADHD symptoms in boys, girls, women, children, and adults. Take tests and learn about treatment options for attention deficit hyperactivity disorder, too. ADHD diagnoses have skyrocketed nearly 50 percent since 2003, bringing the total number of American children with ADHD to nearly 6 million, according to 2015 statistics from the Center for Disease Control and Prevention (CDC).

Children with Attention Deficit Hyperactivity Disorder (ADHD), a condition characterized by inattention, over activity, and impulsivity, are most frequently identified and treated in primary school. Population studies indicate that five percent of children worldwide show impaired levels of attention, as well as hyperactivity. Boys are classified with ADHD approximately twice as frequently as girls and primary school age children approximately twice as frequently as adolescents.

What Is ADHD? Definition & Meaning

Attention deficit hyperactivity disorder (ADHD or ADD) is a complex brain disorder that impacts approximately 11 percent of children aged 4-17 and almost 5 percent of adults in the United States. ADHD is not a behavior disorder. It is a developmental impairment of the brain's self-management system and executive functions.

"ADHD is not a breakdown of the brain in one spot. It's a breakdown in the connectivity, the communication networks, and an immaturity in these networks," says Joel Nigg, Ph.D., professor of psychiatry at Oregon Health & Science University. "These brain networks are interrelated around emotion, attention, behavior, and arousal. People with ADHD have trouble with global self-regulation, not just regulation of attention, which is why there are attentional and emotional issues.

What Are the 3 Types of ADHD

There are three distinct subtypes of ADHD:

• Hyperactive-Impulsive ADHD

• Inattentive ADHD (formerly called ADD)

• Combined ADHD

People with hyperactive-impulsive ADHD act "as if driven by a motor" with little impulse control — moving, squirming impatiently, and interrupting others. People with inattentive ADHD are easily distracted and forgetful. They may be daydreamers who lose track of homework, cell phones, and conversations with regularity.

What Are the Symptoms of ADHD

Common symptoms of ADHD include inattention, lack of focus, poor time management, weak impulse control, exaggerated emotions, hyper focus, hyperactivity, and executive dysfunction.

Doctors diagnose ADHD using symptom criteria from the (DSM-V), which lists nine symptoms that suggest

Inattentive ADHD and nine that suggest Hyperactive-Impulsive ADHD. A child may be diagnosed with ADHD only if he or she exhibits at least six of nine symptoms from the ADHD symptoms and if the symptoms have been noticeable for at least six months in two or more settings for example, at home and at school. What's more, the symptoms must interfere with the child's functioning or development, and at least some of the symptoms must have been apparent before age 12. Older teens and adults may need to consistently demonstrate just five of these symptoms in multiple settings.

ADHD Symptoms in Children

Common Symptoms of Hyperactive-Impulsive ADHD in Children

• Talks excessively and blurts out answers

• Acts as if "driven by a motor"

• Fidgets and squirms in seat constantly

Common Symptoms of Inattentive ADHD in Children

• Distracted or short attention span

• Struggles to organize tasks and activities

• Often loses things and is forgetful

ADHD Symptoms in Adults

Roughly two-thirds of people who experienced ADHD symptoms as a child will continue to experience ADHD symptoms as an adult, though its manifestations change with age.4 What's more, many people with attention deficit were undiagnosed or misdiagnosed as children. They may suffer serious psychological consequences after a lifetime of blaming themselves for ADHD symptoms such as:

• Forgetting names and dates

• Missing deadlines and leaving projects unfinished

• Extreme emotionality and rejection sensitivity

• Becoming easily distracted and disorganized

• Suffering anxiety and depression

What Causes ADHD

ADHD a brain-based, biological disorder. It is not caused by bad parenting, too much sugar, or too many video games. Scientists are investigating whether certain genes, especially ones linked to the neurotransmitter dopamine, play a role in developing ADHD.5 Additional research suggests that exposure to toxins and chemicals may increase a child's risk of having ADHD.

ADHD Diagnosis Information

Any good ADHD diagnosis is based on the criteria defined in the DSM-V. A clinical interview is performed to gather the patient's medical history, and is often supplemented with neuropsychological ADHD tests, which offer greater insight into strengths and weaknesses, and helps identify co morbid (or co-existing) conditions. It can take several hours of talking, test taking, and analysis by an ADHD specialist to diagnose symptoms.

How Is ADHD Diagnosed

Though your child may have some symptoms that seem like ADHD, it might be something else. That's why you need a doctor to check it out.

There is no specific or definitive test for ADHD. Instead, diagnosing is a process that takes several steps and involves gathering a lot of information from multiple sources. You, your child, your child's school, and other caregivers should be involved in assessing your child's behavior. A doctor will also ask what symptoms your child has, how long ago those symptoms started, and how the behavior affects your child and the rest of your family. Doctors diagnose ADHD in children after a child has shown six or more specific symptoms of inattention or hyperactivity on a regular basis for more than 6 months in at least two settings. The doctor will consider how a child's behavior compares with that of other children the same age.

Your child's primary care doctor can determine whether your child has ADHD using standard guidelines developed by the American Academy of Pediatrics, which says the condition may be diagnosed in children ages 4 to 18. Symptoms, though, must begin by age 12.

It is very difficult to diagnose ADHD in children younger than 5. That's because many preschool children have some of the symptoms seen in ADHD in various situations. Also, children change very rapidly during the preschool years.

In some cases, behavior that looks like ADHD might be caused instead by:

- A sudden life change (such asdivorce, a death in the family, or moving)
- Undetected seizures
- Medical disorders affecting brain function
- Anxiety
- Depression
- Bipolar disorder

ADHD Treatment Options

The best ADHD treatment strategies are multimodal ones — combinations of several different, complementary approaches that work together to reduce symptoms. Most ADHD treatment plans include one or more of the following:

ADHD medication including a stimulant like Adderall (amphetamine) or Ritalin (methylphenidate), or a non-stimulant like Strattera or Intuniv

An ADHD diet low in sugar and carbohydrates, and high in protein, greens, and omega-3 fatty acids

ADHD vitamins and supplements particularly zinc, iron, Vitamin C, Vitamin B, and magnesium, which are critical to healthy brain function.

Behavioral Therapy for ADHD, which works best in improving ADHD-associated oppositional behaviors in children, as well as other areas of functioning, like interactions with parents and school, when combined with medication.

ADHD therapies that run the gamut from cognitive behavioral therapy (CBT) and occupational therapy to art or music therapy to play therapy and beyond

Natural remedies for ADHD like mindfulness meditation, brain training, or exercise

How to Find ADHD Doctors

"ADHD is generally ignored in medical education," says William Dodson, M.D., an ADHD specialist and author. "Just 5 years ago, 93 percent of adult psychiatry residencies didn't mention ADHD in four years of training and, amazingly, half of pediatric residencies didn't mention ADHD."

Finding a medical professional who understands ADHD and its comorbid conditions is not easy, but it is vital if you hope to secure an accurate diagnosis and proactive treatment plan. Use these criteria to find an ADHD doctor or other specialist near you.

Can what you eat help attention, focus, or hyperactivity? There's no clear scientific evidence that ADHD is caused by diet or nutritional problems. But certain foods may play at least some role in affecting symptoms in a small group of people, research suggests.

So are there certain things you shouldn't eat if you have the condition? Or if your child has it, should you change what he eats?

Eat Nutritious Food

ADHD diets haven't been researched a lot. Data is limited, and results are mixed. Many health experts, though, think that what you eat and drink may help ease symptoms.

Experts say that whatever is good for the brain is likely to be good for ADHD. You may want to eat:

A high-protein diet. Beans, cheese, eggs, meat, and nuts can be good sources of protein. Eat these kinds of foods in the morning and for after-school snacks. It may improve concentration and possibly make ADHD medications work longer.

More complex carbohydrates. These are the good guys. Load up on vegetables and some fruits, including oranges, tangerines, pears, grapefruit, apples, and kiwi. Eat this type of food in the evening, and it may help you sleep.

More omega-3 fatty acids. You can find these in tuna, salmon, and other cold-water white fish. Walnuts, Brazil nuts, and olive and canola oils are other foods with these in them. You could also take an omega-3 fatty acid supplement. The FDA approved an omega compound called Vayarin as part of an ADHD management strategy.

Foods to Avoid With ADHD

Simple carbohydrates. Cut down on how many of these you eat:

• Candy

• Corn syrup

• Honey

• Sugar

• Products made from white flour

• White rice

• Potatoes without the skins.

Nutritional Supplements for ADHD

Some experts recommend that people with ADHD take a 100% vitamin and mineral supplement each day. Other nutrition experts, though, think that people who eat a normal, balanced diet don't need vitamin or micronutrient supplements. They say there's no scientific evidence that vitamin or mineral supplements help all children who have the disorder.

While a multivitamin may be OK when children, teens, and adults don't eat balanced diets, mega-doses of vitamins can be toxic. Avoid them.

ADHD symptoms vary from person to person. Work with your doctor closely if you're considering taking a supplement.

Elimination Diets for ADHD

To follow one of these, you pick a particular food or ingredient you think might be making your symptoms worse. Then you don't eat anything with that in it. If the symptoms get better or go away, then you keep avoiding that food.

If you cut a food from your diet, can it improve your symptoms? Research in all these areas is ongoing and the results are not clear-cut. Most scientists don't recommend this approach for managing ADHD, though. Still, here are some common areas of concern and what the experts suggest:

Food additives: In 1975, an allergist first proposed that artificial colors, flavors, and preservatives might lead to hyperactivity in some children. Since then, researchers and child behavior experts have hotly debated this issue

ADHD DIET & NUTRITION

Can what you eat help attention, focus, or hyperactivity? There's no clear scientific evidence that ADHD is caused by diet or nutritional problems. But certain foods may play at least some role in affecting symptoms in a small group of people, research suggests.

So are there certain things you shouldn't eat if you have the condition? Or if your child has it, should you change what he eats?

Here are answers to questions about elimination diets, supplements, and foods that may ease symptoms of the disorder.

What Is an ADHD diet

It may include the foods you eat and any nutritional supplements you may take. Ideally, your eating habits would help the brain work better and lessen symptoms, such as restlessness or lack of focus. You may hear about these choices that you could focus on:

• Overall nutrition: The assumption is that some foods you eat may make your symptoms better or worse. You might also not be eating some things that could help make symptoms better.

• Supplementation diet: With this plan, you add vitamins, minerals, or other nutrients. The idea is that it could help you make up for not getting enough of these through what you eat. Supporters of these diets think that if you don't get enough of certain nutrients, it may add to your symptoms.

• Elimination diets: These involve not eating foods or ingredients that you think might be triggering certain behaviors or making your symptoms worse.

Diet Tips and Ideas for Kids with ADHD

Diet and ADHD

Diet hasn't been shown to cause attention-deficit/hyperactivity disorder (ADHD) in children. Additionally, diet alone can't account for the symptoms of ADHD. However, there's no denying that diet plays a crucial role in physical and mental health, especially for growing children.

Children with ADHD have extra challenges. Fueling them with good, nutritious food goes a long way toward helping them cope and stay healthy.

Far too many children aren't getting the vitamins, minerals, and fiber they need. All children require a diet rich in:

- vegetables
- fruits
- whole grains
- protein
- healthy fats
- calcium-rich foods

Such a diet may or may not improve symptoms of ADHD in children, but it will provide them a foundation for good health.

The nutritious diet kids need

Fruits and veggies

Fruits and vegetables provide the vitamins and minerals that growing children need. It also provides them with much needed fiber. Fruit and veggies make a convenient snack food, and they're easy to pack in school lunches. Fruit in particular can satisfy a sweet tooth.

Whole grains

Whole grains are unrefined and contain bran and germ. Whole grains are an excellent source of fiber, plus a variety of other nutrients. Add them to your child's diet through foods such as:

- cereals
- breads
- snack foods

Protein

Protein is important to muscle and tissue growth. Meat is an excellent source for protein. Be sure to choose lean cuts that have low amounts of fat. Avoid processed meats. If you don't want meat in your child's diet or want to reduce their consumption of meat, they can get protein from the following:

• beans

• peas

• nuts

• dairy

Healthy fats

Our bodies need fat, but not all fats are equal. Emphasize the healthy fats, which include monounsaturated fats, polyunsaturated fats, and omega-3 fatty acids. Pick a good selection of foods with healthy fats for your kids from the list below.

Monounsaturated fats

• avocado

• seeds

• nuts

• olives

• canola, olive, and peanut oils

Polyunsaturated fats

• corn

• sesame seeds

- soybeans

- legumes

- safflower and sunflower oils

Omega-3 fatty acids

- herring

- mackerel

- salmon

- sardines

- flaxseeds

- chia seeds

- walnuts

Calcium-rich foods

Calcium is a bone-fortifying mineral that is crucial during early childhood and the adolescent years. This is when bones grow at very fast rates. This essential mineral also plays a role in nerve impulses and hormone production. Calcium is rich in dairy milk, yogurt, and cheese. It's also found in calcium-fortified plant milks such as flax milk, almond milk, and soy milk. Broccoli, beans, lentils, canned fish with bones, and dark leafy greens are plant sources rich in calcium

Foods to avoid

Research has not shown any specific food that causes or cures ADHD. Some foods may affect your child more than others. If you believe a particular food or ingredient aggravates your child's symptoms, eliminate it from their diet to see if it makes a difference.

According to Harvard Medical School, studies show that artificial food coloring may increase hyperactivity in some children. Many foods marketed to children, such as cereals and fruit drinks, use food dyes to make them brightly-colored. Try eliminating these foods from your child's diet and see if their symptoms improve.

According to the Mayo Clinic, the European Union (EU) now requires manufacturers to include a warning on foods with certain additives. The label states that the food may have a negative effect on attention and activity in children.

Studies have not proven that sugar consumption causes hyperactive behavior, according to the American Academy of Pediatrics (AAP). We do know that too much sugar is unhealthy. Evidence that we eat far more sugar than we should is abundant. A study published in JAMA Internal Medicine showed that the average American gets 10 percent of their calories from added sugars. One in 10 Americans gets 25 percent or more of their calories from sugar. Too much sugar contributes to weight gain. In turn this can increase the risk of developing other health problems, such as heart disease and type 2 diabetes.

Other foods that can lead to obesity and high cholesterol include saturated fats, hydrogenated fats, and trans fats. Avoid giving your kids large amounts of foods that contain these fats. Examples include:

Saturated fats

• meat

• poultry

• dairy

Hydrogenated and trans fats

- shortening

- margarine

- packaged snacks

- processed foods

- fast foods

- some frozen pizzas

Fast food and processed foods are generally unhealthy because they contain too much of the following ingredients:

salt

sugar

unhealthy fats

Processed foods in general are very high in calories, and filled with chemical additives and preservatives. They have little or no nutritional value. This type of food fills the belly, but leaves the body wanting.

Medications may cause side effects

ADHD drugs can help improve symptoms by enhancing and balancing neurotransmitters. Neurotransmitters are chemicals that carry signals between neurons in your brain and body. There are several different types of medications used to treat ADHD, including:

stimulants, such as an amphetamine or Adderall (which help you to focus and ignore distractions)

nonstimulants, such as atomoxetine (Strattera) or bupropion (Wellbutrin), can be used if the side effects from stimulants are too much to handle or if other medical conditions prevent use of stimulants

While these drugs can improve concentration, they can also cause some serious potential side effects. Side effects include:

• sleep problems

• mood swings

• loss of appetite

• heart problems

• suicidal thoughts or actions

Not many studies have looked at the long-term effects of these medications. But some research has been done, and it raises red flags. An Australian study published in 2010 found no significant improvement in behavior and attention problems in children between the ages of 5 and 14 years old who took medications for their ADHD. Their self-perception and social functioning didn't improve either.

Instead, the medicated group tended to have higher levels of diastolic blood pressure. They also had slightly lower self-esteem than the non medicated group and performed below age level. The authors of the study emphasized that the sample size and statistical differences were too small to draw conclusions.

1. Forgo food colorings and preservatives

Alternative treatments may help manage some symptoms associated with ADHD, including:

difficulty paying attention

organizational problems

forgetfulness

frequently interrupting

The Mayo Clinic notes that certain food colorings and preservatives may increase hyperactive behavior in some children. Avoid foods with these colorings and preservatives:

sodium benzoate, which is commonly found in carbonated beverages, salad dressings, and fruit juice products

FD&C Yellow No. 6 (sunset yellow), which can be found in breadcrumbs, cereal, candy, icing, and soft drinks

D&C Yellow No. 10 (quinoline yellow), which can be found in juices, sorbets, and smoked haddock

FD&C Yellow No. 5 (tartrazine), which can be found in foods like pickles, cereal, granola bars, and yogurt

FD&C Red No. 40 (allura red), which can be found in soft drinks, children's medications, gelatin desserts, and ice cream

2. Avoid potential allergens

Diets that restrict possible allergens may help improve behavior in some children with ADHD.

It's best to check with an allergy doctor if you suspect that your child has allergies. But you can experiment by avoiding these foods:

chemical additives/preservatives such as BHT (butylated hydroxytoluene) and BHA (butylated hydroxyanisole), which are often used to keep the oil in a product from going bad and can be found in processed food items such as potato chips, chewing gum, dry cake mixes, cereal, butter, and instant mashed potatoes

milk and eggs

chocolate

foods containing salicylates, including berries, chili powder, apples and cider, grapes, oranges, peaches, plums, prunes, and tomatoes (salicylates are chemicals occurring naturally in plants and are the major ingredient in many pain medications)

3. Try EEG biofeedback

Electroencephalographic (EEG) biofeedback is a type of neurotherapy that measures brain waves. A 2011 studyTrusted Source suggested that EEG training was a promising treatment for ADHD.

A child may play a special video game during a typical session. They'll be given a task to concentrate on, such as "keep the plane flying." The plane will start to dive or the screen will go dark if they're distracted. The game teaches the child new focusing techniques over time. Eventually, the child will begin to identify and correct their symptoms.

4. Consider a yoga or tai chi class

Some small studies indicate that yoga may be helpful for people with ADHD. Research published in 2013 Trusted Source reported significant improvements in hyperactivity, anxiety, and social problems in boys with ADHD who practiced yoga regularly.

Some early studies suggest that tai chi also may help improve ADHD symptoms. Researchers found that teenagers with ADHD who practiced tai chi weren't as anxious or hyperactive. They also daydreamed less and displayed fewer inappropriate emotions when they participated in tai chi classes twice a week for five weeks.

5. Spending time outside

Spending time outside may benefit children with ADHD. There is strong evidence that spending even 20 minutes outside can benefit them by improving their concentration. Greenery and nature settings are the most beneficial.

A 2011 study, and several studies before it, supports the claim that regular exposure to outdoors and green space is a safe and natural treatment that can be used to help people with ADHD.

6. Behavioral or parental therapy

For children with more severe cases of ADHD, behavioral therapy can prove beneficial. The American Academy of Pediatrics states that behavioral therapy should be the first step in treating ADHD in young children.

Sometimes called behavioral modification, this approach works on resolving specific problematic behaviors and offers solutions to help prevent them. This can also involve setting up goals and rules for the child. Because behavioral therapy and medication are most effective when used together, it can be a powerful aid in helping your child.

Parental therapy can help provide parents with the tools they need to help their child with ADHD succeed. Equipping parents with techniques and strategies for how to work around behavioral problems can help both the parent and the child in the long term.

What about supplements

Treatment with supplements may help improve symptoms of ADHD. These supplements include:

• zinc

• L-carnitine

• vitamin B-6

• magnesium

However, results have been mixed. Herbs like ginkgo, ginseng, and passionflower may also help calm hyperactivity.

Behavior management plans for children with ADHD

Managing attention deficit hyperactivity disorder (ADHD) in children is about first accepting that your child will behave in challenging ways. But a behavior management plan can make the behavior easier to handle. If you think your child might have attention deficit hyperactivity disorder (ADHD), the first step is to visit your child's GP or pediatrician for further assessment and diagnosis. If your child is diagnosed with ADHD, you and your health professional can work together to develop a behavior management plan.

A behavior management plan guides your child towards appropriate behavior with:

• strategies to encourage good behavior

• social skills to help your child get along with others

• strategies to manage your child's energy levels and tiredness

• strategies to support your child in the classroom

• medication, if your child needs it.

The best plans are usually based on sound professional advice that takes into account what suits your child and family. Plans should consider all aspects of your child's life, including your child's needs and responsibilities at home, at school and in other social settings.

Children with ADHD often experience other difficulties like oppositional defiant disorder or anxiety. You can incorporate strategies to help with these in the management plan.

It's a good idea to discuss your plan with your child's family, careers, therapists and teachers. This helps people have realistic expectations of your child's behaviour. It can also help them understand how best to handle your child's behaviour. And if they have to give your child medication, they'll know how much to give and when.

When you work with health professionals, school teachers, other adults in your child's life, and your family and friends, it can be easier for you and your child to keep to the plan.

Behavior strategies to help children with ADHD

Your child's behavior management plan will probably include strategies that help your child learn the skills she needs to increase cooperative behavior and reduce challenging behavior.

Some simple but effective behavior strategies might include:

• changes to the environment to make it easier for your child to behave well

• clear verbal instructions to help your child understand what you want him to do

• praise for positive behavior to encourage your child to keep behaving well

• predictable daily routines to help your child at demanding times of the day, like when you're getting ready for school and work in the morning.

Social skills to help children with ADHD

Children with attention deficit hyperactivity disorder (ADHD) might need support to get along with other children. So your child's behavior management plan could include some ideas to help your child develop social skills.

These ideas might include:

• rewarding your child for helpful behavior like sharing and being gentle with others

• teaching your child what to do if there's a problem with another child – for example, walking away or talking to a teacher

• teaching your child how to regulate her own behavior – for example, by using a short prompt like 'Stop, think, do'

• helping your child practice social skills by arranging supervised playdates.

Strategies to manage energy and tiredness in children with ADHD

All children find it easier to behave well if they can manage their energy levels and aren't tired, so behavior management plans for attention deficit hyperactivity disorder (ADHD) often cover this.

You can help your child manage energy levels and maintain focus by:

• building rest breaks into activities

• allowing some time for physical exercise breaks while your child is doing learning tasks like reading or homework

• being ready with a few fun but low-key activities like Lego or a puzzle, which your child can do if he starts to get overexcited.

And you can stop your child from getting too tired by:

• getting your child into good sleep habits, like getting to sleep and waking up at about the same time each day

• providing healthy food options for longer-lasting energy and concentration

• making sure your child's screen time is balanced with other activities during the day

• making sure all electronic devices are switched off at least an hour before bed.

Classroom strategies to help children with ADHD

Children with attention deficit hyperactivity disorder (ADHD) can have problems at school. So behaviour management plans should include classroom strategies to support your child's learning.

You could talk with your child's teacher about strategies like:

• dividing tasks into smaller chunks

• offering one-on-one help when possible

• giving your child a 'buddy' who can help her understand what to do

• planning the classroom so your child is seated near the front of the room and away from distractions

• making a visual checklist of tasks that need to be finished or keeping a copy of the school schedule where your child can see it

• doing more difficult learning tasks in the mornings or after breaks

• allowing some extra time to finish tasks.

To get the support your child needs for learning, language and physical problems at school, you might need to advocate for your child. This could involve talking to your child's classroom teacher, the principal or the additional needs support officer about special programs, funding and other help for your child.

Schools can help by setting out support plans in an individual learning plan for your child. The school should also work with you to set and review your child's learning goals regularly.

ADHD medications

If your child needs medication to help him manage his attention deficit hyperactivity disorder (ADHD), this will be included in his behaviour management plan.

Stimulant medications

Doctors will sometimes prescribe stimulant medications for children diagnosed with ADHD. These medications improve the way the parts of the brain 'talk' to each other. This can help children with attention and self-regulation.

Methylphenidate is the most commonly used medication of this type. It's sold under the brand names Ritalin 10, Ritalin LA and Concerta. These different medications release the methylphenidate at different rates and different times of the day.

Other stimulant medications are dexamphetamine or lisdexamfetamine. Lisdexamfetamine is sold under the brand name Vyvanse.

Your child's paediatrician or psychiatrist will be able to work out which drug and dose will be right for your child.

Here are a few questions you might want to ask your doctor:

• How long will each dose last?

• What are the side effects of the medication?

• How will the medication be monitored?

• How long will my child stay on medication?

Non-stimulant medication

There are also some non-stimulant medications available for treating ADHD. These include Strattera (atomoxetine), Catapres (clonidine) and Intuniv (guanfacine). These medications can help to reduce anxiety too.

Side effects of ADHD medications

These medications can cause some side effects – for example, loss of appetite, which can affect your child's weight gain or growth. Other side effects might include difficulty getting to sleep, tummy upsets or headaches.

Because of these possible side effects, a child who has been prescribed medication should always be closely monitored by a health professional.

Most side effects are mild and don't last long. If there are side effects that don't go away, your health professional might change the dose or timing of medication, or suggest trying a different medication.

Treatments that are backed up by science are most likely to work, be worth your time, money and energy, and be safe for your child. If you're interested in other ADHD treatments, it's always a good idea to speak with a health professional about them.

looking after yourself

Looking after yourself by asking for help and support is a big part of managing your child's attention deficit hyperactivity disorder (ADHD). Here are some options for you to think about:

• Ask for help from family members and friends. If your child relates well to a particular family member, like an aunt or grandparent, that person might be able to help in difficult situations like shopping, or spend some time with your child while you get some chores done.

• Speak to your child's teacher about classroom behavior strategies that you can try out at home.

• Go to a support group for parents of children with ADHD.

• Talk to your child's health professional about any difficulties you're having.

• Learn about stress and how you can handle it.

ADHD diet plan and recipe

Diet hasn't been shown to cause attention-deficit/hyperactivity disorder (ADHD) in children. Additionally, diet alone can't account for the symptoms of ADHD. However, there's no denying that diet plays a crucial role in physical and mental health, especially for growing children.

Children with ADHD have extra challenges. Fueling them with good, nutritious food goes a long way toward helping them cope and stay healthy. Far too many children aren't getting the vitamins, minerals, and fiber they need. All children require a diet rich in:

• vegetables

• fruits

• whole grains

• protein

• healthy fats

• calcium-rich foods

Such a diet may or may not improve symptoms of ADHD in children, but it will provide them a foundation for good health.

The nutritious diet kids need

Fruits and veggies

Fruits and vegetables provide the vitamins and minerals that growing children need. It also provides them with much needed fiber. Fruit and veggies make a convenient snack food, and they're easy to pack in school lunches. Fruit in particular can satisfy a sweet tooth.

Whole grains

Whole grains are unrefined and contain bran and germ. Whole grains are an excellent source of fiber, plus a variety of other nutrients. Add them to your child's diet through foods such as:

• cereals

• breads

• snack foods

Protein

Protein is important to muscle and tissue growth. Meat is an excellent source for protein. Be sure to choose lean cuts that have low amounts of fat. Avoid processed meats. If you don't want meat in your child's diet or want to reduce their consumption of meat, they can get protein from the following:

• beans

• peas

• nuts

• dairy

Healthy fats

Our bodies need fat, but not all fats are equal. Emphasize the healthy fats, which include monounsaturated fats, polyunsaturated fats, and omega-3 fatty acids. Pick a good selection of foods with healthy fats for your kids from the list below.

Monounsaturated fats

• avocado

• seeds

• nuts

• olives

• canola, olive, and peanut oils

Polyunsaturated fats

• corn

• sesame seeds

• soybeans

• legumes

• safflower and sunflower oils

Omega-3 fatty acids

• herring

- mackerel

- salmon

- sardines

- flaxseeds

- chia seeds

- walnuts

Calcium-rich foods

Calcium is a bone-fortifying mineral that is crucial during early childhood and the adolescent years. This is when bones grow at very fast rates. This essential mineral also plays a role in nerve impulses and hormone production. Calcium is rich in dairy milk, yogurt, and cheese. It's also found in calcium-fortified plant milks such as flax milk, almond milk, and soy milk. Broccoli, beans, lentils, canned fish with bones, and dark leafy greens are plant sources rich in calcium.

Foods to avoid

Research has not shown any specific food that causes or cures ADHD. Some foods may affect your child more than others. If you believe a particular food or ingredient aggravates your child's symptoms, eliminate it from their diet to see if it makes a difference.

According to Harvard Medical School, studies show that artificial food coloring may increase hyperactivity in some children. Many foods marketed to children, such as cereals and fruit drinks, use food dyes to make them brightly-colored. Try eliminating these foods from your child's diet and see if their symptoms improve.

According to the Mayo Clinic, the European Union (EU) now requires manufacturers to include a warning on foods with certain additives. The label states that the food may have a negative effect on attention and activity in children.

Studies have not proven that sugar consumption causes hyperactive behavior, according to the American Academy of Pediatrics (AAP). We do know that too much sugar is unhealthy. Evidence that we eat far more sugar than we should is abundant. A study published in JAMA Internal Medicine showed that the average American gets 10 percent of their calories from added sugars. One in 10 Americans gets 25 percent or more of their calories from sugar. Too much sugar contributes to weight gain. In turn this can increase the risk of developing other health problems, such as heart disease and type 2 diabetes.

Other foods that can lead to obesity and high cholesterol include saturated fats, hydrogenated fats, and trans fats. Avoid giving your kids large amounts of foods that contain these fats. Examples include:

Saturated fats

• meat

• poultry

• dairy

Hydrogenated and trans fats

• shortening

• margarine

• packaged snacks

• processed foods

• fast foods

• some frozen pizzas

Fast food and processed foods are generally unhealthy because they contain too much of the following ingredients:

• salt

• sugar

• unhealthy fats

Processed foods in general are very high in calories, and filled with chemical additives and preservatives. They have little or no nutritional value. This type of food fills the belly, but leaves the body wanting.

Smart snacking

Instead of this Choose this

• prepackaged fruit-flavored snacks • real fruit, such as apples, oranges, bananas, pears, nectarines, plums, raisins, grapes

• homemade fruit smoothie

• dried fruit

• potato chips and other crunchy munchies • pan-popped popcorn, with little or no butter and salt

• baked whole-grain chips or pretzels

• diced carrots and celery, with hummus

• broccoli and cauliflower, with fresh salsa or yogurt dip

• roasted chickpeas

• ice cream • yogurt

• cut up watermelon and cantaloupe, or other fruit mixture

• homemade fruit smoothies

• candy bars, cookies, and other sweets • dried fruit and nut mixture

• dark chocolate covered fruit

• popular kiddie cereals • whole-grain, high fiber cereal, with fresh berries and nuts

• instant oatmeal packets with added sugars • plain oatmeal, with bananas, berries, or stone fruit

More dietary tips

Most children benefit from routine. For a child with ADHD a routine is especially helpful. Schedule regular meal and snack times, if you can. Try not to let your child go for more than a few hours without eating. Too much time between meals and snacks may lead to overindulging later.

Avoid fast food restaurants and junk food aisles in the grocery store. One of the reasons we eat so many bad foods is because they're easy to access. To eliminate the temptation, don't keep junk foods in your home. Stock plenty of fruits and veggies to satisfy growling stomachs in a pinch.

If your child is used to eating a lot of bad food, change won't come easily. It takes some time for children to connect dietary changes to feeling healthier.

Ask your child's doctor if you should give them a multivitamin or other nutritional supplements. A dietitian can also help you get your family's eating habits on the right track.

The takeaway

Healthy dietary habits begin in childhood and can last a lifetime. Children with ADHD are no exception to this rule. They too should maintain a well-balanced healthy diet. Research has not shown any specific food to cause or cure ADHD in children, But as with all kids, its best to avoid excessive amounts of sugar, salt, and unhealthy fats.

One of the most important things you can do is set a good example. Make sure your own diet is healthy. Your children depend on you to provide the meals and snacks they need to make it through the day. Make healthy choices and use these tips to keep your kid healthy while coping with ADHD.

9 Healthy Food Rules for ADHD Families: What to Eat, What to Avoid

Healthy food is so powerful. A well-rounded diet can have a powerful, positive effect on your cognition, mood, memory, and behavior. The wrong diet can aggravate ADHD symptoms. Here's what you should (and absolutely should not) be eating to help your brain and body.

Healthy Food for ADHD Brains

The right foods can have a powerful, positive effect on your cognition, mood, memory, and behavior. The wrong foods can worsen symptoms of attention deficit disorder (ADHD or ADD). That's why it's important to note the best foods for ADHD.

In two studies done in Holland, Lidy Pelsser, Ph.D., demonstrated that an elimination diet (eliminating sugar, gluten, dairy, eggs, certain meats, and food dyes) improved symptoms in 70 percent of children with ADHD. (That was without eating some of the best foods for ADHD, the powerful brain-focusing foods that I will tell you about later.) As someone who knows what it's like to grow up in an ADHD household filled with drama, this little food fact got my attention.

Everything you put on the end of your fork matters. When you eat to improve your health, you improve the quality of your life. Food impacts neurotransmitter levels of serotonin and dopamine, which play a big role in how you feel and perceive the world. Serotonin, for instance, is responsible for mood, sleep regulation, and appetite control.

When levels of this neurotransmitter drop, the results can be mood disorders, anxiety, and negativity. This may be why we crave carbohydrates such as pasta, bread, and chocolate, all of which raise serotonin levels temporarily. Complex carbs, such as apples and sweet potatoes, work the same magic, but don't set you up for more cravings.

Likewise, dopamine helps to increase focus and motivation. Eating small amounts of protein throughout the day can boost dopamine and stabilize blood sugar.

It is critical to make sure that the food you eat is loaded with nutrients that your body is able to properly digest and absorb. At the Amen Clinic, we created nine simple food guidelines to help you heal your brain and body.

Rule 1: Eat high-quality calories, but not too many.

The quality of your food affects how your brain and body work. Try to eat high-quality food, and be careful with calories. Impulsivity leads many people diagnosed with ADHD to eat the wrong things too often. In fact, impulsivity is associated with unhealthy weight gain, which has been shown to be bad for the brain. Eat only high-quality calories. One cinnamon roll contains 720 calories and a small quiche more than 1,000 calories while a 400-calorie salad made of spinach, salmon, blueberries, apples, walnuts, and red bell peppers will increase your energy and, maybe, make you smarter.

It's not as simple as calories in, calories out. Some calories adversely affect your hormones, your taste buds, and your health. Eating sugar and processed food, even in small amounts, leads to craving more food and feeling less energetic. You can eat more if you eat healthy, high-quality food that gives you energy and turns on the hormones that affect metabolism.

Rule 2: Drink plenty of water.

Your brain is 80 percent water. Anything that dehydrates it, such as too much caffeine or alcohol, impairs your cognition and judgment. Drink plenty of water every day.

To know whether you are drinking enough water for your brain, a good general rule is to drink half your weight in ounces per day. If you are significantly obese, don't drink more than 120 ounces a day. If you are an athlete, make sure to replenish electrolytes after the game or working out. Cutting out sugary drinks and juice eliminates about 400 calories a day from the average American diet. That allows you to either eat more healthy food or eliminates a lot of calories, if you are trying to shed pounds.

Rule 3: Eat high-quality, lean protein.

It is important to start each day with protein to boost your focus and concentration. Protein helps balance your blood sugar, increases focus, and gives your brain the necessary building blocks for brain health. Think of it as medicine, and take it in small doses. Recent studies3 show that consuming large amounts of protein at one time can cause oxidative stress (a problem that burdens your body and brain), making you feel sick.

Great sources of protein include wild fish, skinless turkey or chicken, beans (eat them like a condiment, not too often or too much), raw nuts, and vegetables such as broccoli and spinach. I use spinach instead of lettuce in my salads for a nutrition boost. Protein powders can also be a good source, but read the labels. Whey protein contains casein, which is an excitotoxin in the brain, and can be overly stimulating for some people. Many companies put sugar and other unhealthful ingredients in their powders. My personal preference is pea and rice protein blends.

Rule 4: Eat smart carbs.

Eat carbohydrates that do not spike your blood sugar and are high in fiber, such as those found in vegetables and fruits, like blueberries and apples. Carbohydrates are not the enemy; they are essential to your health. Bad carbohydrates — ones that have been stripped of nutritional value, such as sugar and simple carbs — are the problem.

Sugar is not your friend. It increases inflammation in your body (which leads to inflammation in the brain, as well) and erratic brain cell firing. Sugar gets you hooked, and perhaps plays a role in aggression. In a recent study, children who were given sugar every day showed a significantly higher risk for violence later in life. The less sugar in your life, the better your life will be.

Get to know the Glycemic Index (GI). It rates carbohydrates according to their effects on blood sugar. Carbs are ranked on a scale of one to 100+ (glucose is 100). Low-glycemic foods, as you would imagine, have a lower number. This means they do not spike your blood sugar, and are generally healthier for you. High-glycemic foods have a higher number; they quickly elevate your blood sugar, and are not as healthy for you. In general, I like to stay with foods that have a GI rating under 60.

Eating a diet that is filled with low-glycemic foods will lower your blood glucose levels, decrease cravings, and help you focus.

When eating carbs, choose those that are high in fiber. Experts recommend eating 25 to 35 grams of fiber a day, but studies suggest that most people fall short of that. Boost your fiber by eating lots of vegetables and a little fruit. Think of legumes as you would a condiment. You can add fiber to smoothies, but don't use grain-based fiber. My favorite types of fiber supplements are inulin or glucomannan. When reading a food label, you want to look for more than 5 grams of fiber and fewer than 5 grams of sugar per serving.

Rule 5: Focus on healthy fats.

Good fats are essential to your health. Essential fatty acids are called "essential" for a reason. The solid weight of your brain is 60 percent fat (after all the water is removed).

When the medical establishment recommended that we eliminate fat from our diets, we got fat.

You want to eliminate bad fats from your meals — trans fats, fried fats, and fat from cheaply raised, industrially farmed animals that are fed corn and soy. Fats found in pizza, ice cream, and cheeseburgers fool the brain into ignoring the signals that tell your brain that you are full. They disrupt the hormones that send those signals to your brain. Focus on healthy fats, especially those that contain omega-3 fatty acids, found in foods like salmon, sardines, avocados, walnuts, chia seeds, and dark green leafy vegetables.

Rule 6: Eat from the rainbow.

Eat foods that reflect the colors of the rainbow, such as blueberries, pomegranates, yellow squash, and red bell peppers. They boost the antioxidant levels in your body and help keep your brain young.

I'm not talking about Skittles, jelly beans, or M&Ms. Nor do I mean grape jelly, mustard (which contains food dye and sometimes gluten), or ketchup, which is loaded with sugar. These highly processed, sugar-filled foods have no place in your pantry if you are trying to use food to heal your brain.

Rule 7: Cook with herbs and spices.

Some herbs and spices are so powerful that you could keep them in your medicine cabinet instead of your kitchen cabinet.

• Turmeric, found in curry, contains a chemical that has been shown to decrease the plaque in the brain thought to be responsible for Alzheimer's disease.

• In several studies, a saffron extract was found to be as effective as antidepressant medication.

• Scientific evidence has shown that rosemary, thyme, and sage help boost memory.

• Cinnamon has been shown to help improve attention and blood sugar regulation.It is high in antioxidants and is a natural aphrodisiac.

• Garlic and oregano boost blood flow to the brain.

• The hot spicy taste of ginger, cayenne, and black pepper comes from gingerols, capsaicin, and piperine, compounds that help boost metabolism

Rule 8: Make sure your food is clean.

Whenever you can, eat organically grown or raised foods. Pesticides used in commercial farming can accumulate in your brain and body, even though the levels in each food may be low. Also, eat hormone-free, antibiotic-free meat from animals that are free-range and grass-fed. Grass-fed bison and beef are 30 percent lower in palmitic acid the saturated fat associated with heart disease than industrially raised beef (fed corn, soy, and pharmaceuticals, and restricted in movement).

It is critical to know and understand what you are eating. You are not only what you eat, you are also what the animals you eat ate. In addition, eliminate food additives, preservatives, and artificial dyes and sweeteners. To do so, start reading food labels. If you do not know what is in a food item or product, don't eat it. Would you buy something if you did not know how much it cost?

Fish is a great source of healthy protein and fat, but it is important to know about the mercury levels in fish. Here are a couple of general rules to guide you:

1) The larger the fish, the more mercury it probably contains, so go for smaller varieties.

2) From the safe fish choices, eat a variety of fish, preferably those highest in omega-3s, like wild Alaskan salmon, sardines, anchovies, and Pacific halibut.

Be mindful of pesticide levels in fruits and vegetables. Foods with the highest levels are: celery, peaches, apples, blueberries, sweet bell peppers, cucumbers, cherries, collard greens, kale, grapes, green beans, strawberries, nectarines, spinach, potatoes.

Foods with the lowest levels of pesticide residues are: onions, pineapple, sweet peas (frozen), cabbage, mushrooms, eggplant, avocado, kiwi fruit, broccoli, watermelon, cantaloupe, sweet corn (frozen), asparagus, bananas, papaya, grapefruit.

Rule 9: Eliminate problem foods.

If you're having trouble with focus, mood, energy, memory, weight, blood sugar, or blood pressure, eliminate the foods that might be causing trouble, especially wheat and any other gluten-containing grain or food, dairy, soy, and corn.

Did you know that gluten makes some people emotionally unstable? There are reports of people having psychotic episodes when they're exposed to gluten. When these people eliminate wheat and other gluten sources, their stomachs and brains function better.

We have many stories of patients who lose weight and improve symptoms of brain fog, irritability, eczema, and irritable bowel syndrome when they eliminate gluten from their diet.

One of our patients became violent whenever he ate MSG. What's worse, MSG is not required to be listed on a label unless it is a single food additive. It can be disguised by being added in with other ingredients.

Children with ADHD and autism often feel and behave better when we put them on elimination diets that get rid of wheat, dairy, processed foods, sugar and sugar alternatives, food dyes, and additives

ADD ADHD Recipes for Attention Deficit Kids

Breakfast

Here are some easy breakfasts that you can make for your kids.

Eggs scrambled in low fat butter and a glass of orange juice. Also add a piece of toast with all natural jam.

Slice of whole-grain bread toasted with a little whipped butter or margarine and a dab of all-fruit jam; low-fat milk.

Whole grain bread dipped in egg and toasted in a skillet. Then served with a sugar free syrup and low fat butter. Also a little pan seared thin ham on the side.

Whole-grain cereal with low-fat or 2% milk with some lean meat like a pork chop, chicken or steak. Add some orange pieces or orange juice.

Plain yogurt mixed with fresh fruit like apples or mandarin oranges.

Homemade Instant Breakfast Smoothie and a sausage patty. Smoothie can include milk, some frozen yogurt, fresh bananas, other fruit like strawberries and a protein supplement if desired.

Mixed nuts; fruit; glass of low-fat milk.

Lunch

Grilled-cheese sandwich made with whole-grain bread and two-percent cheese; glass of orange juice.

Natural peanut butter on whole-grain bread, with a dab of all-fruit jam.

Shakes and Smoothies

Shakes and smoothies are a great way to blend together a variety of great ingredients into one healthy drink. Here are some sample recipes.

Fruit Smoothie #1

- 4 ounces of whole or 2% milk

- 4 ounces of frozen yogurt
- 3-4 tablespoons protein powder
- 1/2 cup bananas, blueberries, strawberries, or peach slices. Fresh is best but frozen is fine also.
- Ice
- Mix these ingredients in a blender, add ice and blend until smooth. Serve with whole grain toast and sausage patty if desired.

Mocha Latte Protein Shake #1

- Cup of Coffee
- Cup of Milk
- 1 tablespoon protein powder
- Pack of Splenda
- Cocoa Powder
- Ice
- Pour the ingredients into a blender and blend until smooth. This protein shake tastes good and can helpful in improving focus and concentration. Since 100 milligrams of caffeine is about the same as a 5 milligram dose of ritalin this drink often

makes a good substitute. You can vary the ingredients a little to your childs taste.

Keep in mind that some people have issues with caffeine, however, for most people this recipe is helpful and boosts focus for an hour or two. Use your own discretion. The protein helps to fuel the body and brain. Try a shake or two and if they work have one at breakfast and maybe at lunch. Leave plenty of time to let the caffeine get out of the childs system before bed.

Fruit Smoothie #2

- 4 ounces of whole milk
- 4 ounces of vanilla frozen yogurt
- 1 tablespoon flax seed oil
- 3-4 tablespoons protein powder
- 3/4 cup fresh or frozen fruit
- Ice
- Mix these ingredients in a blender, add ice and blend until smooth. Flax seed oil is felt to be beneficial in treating ADHD.

Brain Boost Omega 3 Smoothie

- 2 cups Ice Cold Pineapple Juice
- 2 Tablespoons Flax Oil
- 2 Tablespoons Protein Powder
- 4 Tablespoons Plain or Vanilla Yogurt
- 2 Cups Frozen Strawberries
- Ice
- Combine all ingredients in a blender and puree to a smooth consistency. Add ice cubes as desired to put the "frozen" in this frozen yogurt smoothie. Enjoy!

Tropical Strawberry Smoothie

- 1/2 Cup Pineapple
- 1/2 Cup Peaches
- 1/2 Cup Strawberries
- 1/2 Cup Frozen Yogurt
- 1 Teaspoon Flaxseed Oil
- Ice
- Blend ingredients together unil smooth.

Made in the USA
Middletown, DE
30 January 2021